Co-published by Okay Then and Madbooks
Pittsburgh, PA
© 2024, Hanna du Plessis
Illustrations by Hanna du Plessis
ISBN 979-8-9902509-3-2

First edition, 2024
okaythen.net/books

# Bedsores and Bliss

Finding Fullness of Life
with a Terminal Diagnosis

Hanna du Plessis

Okay Then | Office of
Stubborn
Gladness

Mad Books
Carlow University

This little book is about journey. How do we keep walking and finding our way when the road ahead must pass through difficulty? This question feels relevant to where we are globally. As things we once depended on unravel, die or disappear, when we are hurting, how do we keep going?

Hanna du Plessis, August 2024

# Timeline

| | |
|---|---|
| November 2022 | Friend: "You should see a doctor." |
| January 2023 | "It's looking like ALS." |
| March | "You have ALS." |
| June | Writing residency in Ireland |
| | Life goes on, symptoms progress |
| January 2024 | Writing residency in Pittsburgh |
| March - August | Life goes on, symptoms progress |

# Contents

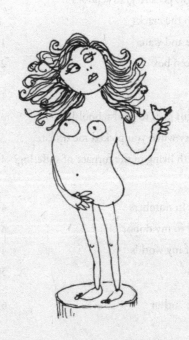

# The question

I am embarrassed to say I didn't notice the symptoms. Friends did. Well that is not entirely true. I did notice that I had little energy. But since burnout is nothing new to me, I thought it was that—me "not setting firm enough boundaries," or me "caring for others at the expense of myself."

I was working full time, running workshops on social change while teaching part time in New York City. I spent time in my community and with my partner and his children. I took a writing workshop at Carlow University. I swam and did yoga.

When my speech started to slur, I thought it was my cold mixed with my tired. But my colleague

1

pulled me aside and said, "I am concerned about your speech. I think you should see a doctor." Then it hit me.

*Something might be wrong.*

I lived with the knowledge that I might have a serious neurological disease for five months before I was able to see the ALS specialist. The day I am diagnosed, the specialist says,

"This is the most terrible disease.
Something you do not wish
on your worst enemy."

This. This body unhurriedly paralyzing itself over years.

He tells me I have ALS—Amyotrophic Lateral Sclerosis. A "bulbar-onset" case, which begins with slurred speech and trouble swallowing. It progresses faster than limb-onset ALS, and most people die within two years of diagnosis.

I ask him,

*"Is life with ALS worth living?"*

In my journal I write,

"I am forty-six. I have my life ahead of me. I have broken out of the cycle of survival. I am coming into my own as an artist. For the first time since arriving in the US fourteen years ago, I have work that I love, which pays enough for me to indulge in pleasure. I can take a week-long textile printing workshop, indigo dye over my eager hands. I can disappear into Utah's slot canyons with my new and gorgeous family. And I no longer feel like an immigrant outsider. I participate in a vibrant community. I crave living! Performing, publishing, collaborating, exhibiting, traveling, teaching, nesting, seeing the kids through school, caring for my people and my aging parents. My family lives till they are toothless.

I cannot be dying.
Not when I am only starting to live."

# A dying girl goes to grad school I

May 31, 2023

Dear Future Ireland Companions,
I feel both excited and shaky to join you next week. Excited because it's going to be more than wonderful. And shaky because I am not in good health. I have bulbar onset ALS. The good news is that I am only seven months in, so my body still functions relatively well. The bad news is that I don't function as I would like to, and it feels scary to venture out of my familiar circle. Hence, I am writing to tell you what you might expect and to ask for your companionship in this strange time of living within a dying body.

**Speaking and breathing**

Participating in conversation helps me feel vital and alive, but it's becoming much more difficult to speak. Not only are the muscles in my mouth and throat atrophying, but my lungs have also lost 30% of their capacity due to my waning diaphragm. I am enlisting technology – an app on my phone that will speak for me (in the voice of a terribly uptight South African lady!), a speaker to help you hear me if we're in a crowd, a board to write on, and maybe I'll bring my ventilator to class. My ask is that you talk to me normally even though I don't sound normal. Please make space for my contributions. If I or anyone falls silent for a while, please ask us what we're thinking.

Getting COVID can be dangerous in my condition, so I'll mask up as much as my lungs will allow me. Thank you also for being COVID careful.

**Use of hands and feet**

Simple things like opening a water bottle or cutting celery is becoming too difficult for me, and I might ask for assistance. I can also spill a cup of something if I sneeze. Because some of my muscles are dying, the rest need to work so much harder, so I get tired quickly. And I used to hike a lot and I wish to see some of the world with you! This might mean using a wheelchair (which I've never done!), so, let's see how that's going to feel for us all. I don't want to hold you back, and I want to gift myself the experience of being there.

## Eating and swallowing

Eh! This is the hardest part for me! I grew up with a Swiss-German dad and was sent to etiquette school. And here I am now with mud-mouth and the three cousins:

### MUD-MOUTH

Often there is food stuck in my teeth and my tongue can't reach it, so I don't know. Please signal for me to get that spinach out!

The following three are cousins:

### GROSS THROAT

Sometimes I really need to work at clearing my throat or soft palate and that might sound excessive or irritating.

### CHOKE-CHAMPION

I am developing super choking abilities where I can involuntarily choke on my own saliva and anything else liquid!

VESUVIUS

This is my worst fear, people. That I might have liquid in my mouth and then either choke or laugh so that the liquid comes flying out.

My ask for the three cousins is that you just be with me as if it's normal, or if you have it in you, join me in making strange noises and gestures so it becomes more of a communal game and less of an individual shame.

Thank you for reading this. Going on a writing retreat like this has always been a dream of mine and I'm so glad I get to share this with you.

With excitement and gratitude,
Hanna

# Caught in
# the cracks

I have landed in a seam, in the crack between two airlines. One who has done their duty and has no further responsibility toward me, and one who has not yet taken custody of me.

> I take my place
>     on the fake leather seat
>         in Terminal A
> and watch my mind
>     throw a temper tantrum.

***

I've never before attempted international travel while terminally ill. This trip, a ten-day residency in Dublin, is part of my post diagnosis choice to enroll in grad school, a defiant stance in the face of a terminal disease. I like leaving for a trip, but this time I like it even more because I'm leaving behind the many reminders of my illness and of a future I still grapple to embrace:

- The five boxes of horrid tasting medication I start when I return from my trip

- The walker I use outside

- The slanted stacks of papers from the medical maze

- The unopened and unassembled shower chair for when standing showers become too difficult

- The plastic arm to help the ventilator pipe fit onto a wheelchair.

This trip marks the first time I use a wheelchair to travel. Surely this is not my first time being wheeled around. I've been in strollers, on bike handlebars, in wheelbarrows. But now it is my adult independent self that is asked to sit and be moved by someone else.

9

I have come to know the travel terrain. I know how to find my way sure-footedly. I can even approach a hostile immigration counter and hand over my "green mamba"—a term South Africans use to describe our passports. But now my sure-footedness has been replaced by the feeling of being on ice skates with no rail in sight.

\*\*\*

I didn't book my tickets for this trip, the school booked them for me. I fly from Pittsburgh to Philadelphia, have a six-hour layover, and then depart for Dublin, our final destination. They put me on the same flight as Donna, another Carlow student. Donna has booked a lounge suite where we can pass the time during the layover.

I don't know Donna, but anticipating her presence offers me a reprieve from my fears. On my last flight, when the cabin's oxygen level dropped, my compromised lungs anxiously sucked air in like a flailing fish out of water. I panicked. At least I now had my ventilator and Donna could help me get it out of the overhead compartment, as my arms have become too weak to lift it myself. If we can work through the breathing thing and TSA doesn't confiscate my medical meal supplement, I'll be fine. My hope for the trip takes the form of a small prayer, "Please get me there safely."

After check-in and a last long lean into my mother's arms, my body buckles into a wheelchair. For a moment I want to brace—fasten a seatbelt or hold the handlebars. But Kim—the airport employee who guides my chair through the terminal—pushes just slowly enough for me to trust the ride.

My beautiful body reads the different floor textures like braille. The coaster-sized porcelain tiles with their wide lines of grout reverberate like cobblestones. The expansion joints in the terrazzo floor are so delicate, I need to listen with my entirety to feel them. The aluminum plates that hide underfloor cables make for hiccups in the ride. And the rug feels soft, almost like sand slowing us down.

At the gate they need me to check my carry-on, but my ventilator is in it. "Take the ventilator out," they say, "and then check the bag."

"No," I say, "the ventilator pipes are too fragile and will get damaged in my soft-shell bag."

"Okay, okay. You can have it on the plane."

Thank goodness I can still speak.

After we disembark in Philly, I see Donna only briefly. The airline has checked her bag through from Pittsburgh to Dublin. But they told me that they couldn't book mine through in the same way. I must pick it up in Philly baggage claim during the layover, then recheck it to Dublin. With a wheelchair.

\*\*\*

This is how I've come to be left in the seam of Terminal A, waiting in a crack between flights, wondering how other people manage this. I am hot and sweaty, and I am well positioned for a temper tantrum. It's nap time, I've not had lunch, I am thirsty and tired. If you have ALS, it is important that you rest, hydrate and eat regularly. I can't wait to check this bag, slip through security to food, naps and water.

The airline that must check my bag to Dublin won't open for two-and-a-half hours. The terminal is a single room, with no bathroom and nowhere to buy food.

I was deposited in this crack in Terminal A by Breeze, the airline attendant who meets me when I disembark in Philly, and whose responsibility it is to ferry me through the airport until my next flight. Together, it seems we have been through quite a journey, that goes something like this:

We get my bag at the luggage claim and take it to Aer Lingus.

"Oh no, sorry," they say. "This ticket is two separate bookings. We can't check your bag, you must go to Terminal A."

Breeze whisks me away and suddenly we are at security. "Shouldn't we go to Terminal A first?" I ask.

"We're going there," she replies. I am confused. In my mind you check your bag before you go through security.

TSA screens my large bag, the one I am planning to check. A blonde guy with blue gloves works his way through my belongings, and I feel angry as he unwraps my stuff, opens my candle and smells it. He takes out the protein powders to screen them. Sets aside my protein shakes and takes apart my blender.

"But I want to check the bag, not take it on the plane," I say, confused.

"But you can't take these through security."

I don't *want* to go through security. I just want to check my darn bag and then go through security without it. Another lady jumps into our confusion and amplifies it with unsolicited advice. My eyes burn with frustration, and simultaneously I feel ashamed that something so small can make this white lady cry.

"Are you okay?" asks Breeze.

"Yes, yes," I say.

TSA Man says it again. "Either leave the shakes

and blender here, or go back and check your bag."

We turn around to go to Terminal A without going through security. "How do we get there?" I ask.

"We walk," Breeze replies. Walking turns out to be a rotten task with me, two bags on my lap and Breeze—weighing no more than a suitcase herself—tries to push me in an old wheelchair while also dragging my 46-pound bag behind her.

"Wait Breeze," I say. "I can walk. Let's work this out." I get up and push my carry-on bags perched on the wheelchair. Breeze brings the large bag. If I had studied Philly's airport, I would have known that Terminal A is annoyingly far from Terminal F and that a shuttle would have been a smarter plan. Maybe not for a fit self, but definitely for this self! I stop a couple of times to catch my breath.

When we finally arrive at Terminal A is when we receive the news: it will be two and a half hours until I can do anything else in service to this mission. Since Breeze and I can think of no other practical option, she leaves the wheelchair with me and goes on with her day.

The first airline's job to hand me over to the next airline is done.

Here I sit.

\*\*\*

If I was able-bodied I would find a way out of here to food and water, at least. But I am not. Our world is not set up to take genuine care. The first airline, knowing of my condition, hearing my request to book my bag through to Dublin and my need for a wheelchair, did not think in terms of care. Even though checking a bag all the way through was possible—my travel companion with the exact same travel plan had done just that—Breeze (an employee of that airline) was not empowered to think strategically with me.

What is the impact of landing in this unsupported and unseen no-mans-land? The lack of water makes my mucus thick so I can gag on it. It worsens the fasciculations in my body, making it harder to sleep. And contributes to constipation and ass-figs (also known as hemorrhoids). My body hopefully meets its need for protein and calories by taking from my belly fat rather than muscles or organs. My tiredness will be passed onto my future self. (And it was. I was so exhausted upon arrival that I could hardly muster the energy to chew my sandwich.)

All of this is manageable. At least this time and for this person. But what about all the others who have slipped through the cracks?

Once I stood in front of a glass case in the national history museum of Mexico, looking at a figure carved out of rock. The description said that once very, very, very long ago, people who were born with Down's Syndrome were considered gods. Imagine that!

Imagine if tomorrow everyone on
the margins woke with garlands
of flowers and prayers and incense
around them.

Imagine their joy as they stepped
or rolled or stumbled into a world
so tightly woven together in
reverence for life that they never
feared slipping through the cracks
ever again.

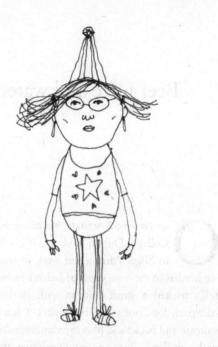

# Beet juice and water

Our two-week writers' residency at Trinity College Dublin ended with a weekend in Sligo. After a full week of workshops, we headed to the west coast of Ireland by bus. Most folks packed a small suitcase with clothes and a backpack for books and computers. I too had my suitcase and backpack, plus my ventilator case, a bag with ventilator pipes and my humidifier and a fifth bag with my protein powder, smoothie ingredients and blender.

Thankfully Rachel, a longtime assistant to the program, came over to help me pack,
as everything is more difficult
with weakening hands and
a careful-not-to-fall walk.

She helped me carry my bags. For a moment I stood in front of the Graduates Memorial Building surrounded by my five bags, feeling the afternoon sun and the solid granite steps. And then, like ants carrying cookie crumbs, my new friends whisked my bags to the bus stop.

The same kind hands repeated this when we arrived at Saint Angela's College. Everyone settled in, then went into town for dinner. But after a morning of class and a four-hour bus ride I did not have the energy to go. So I stayed in. My room had a view of the lake. The sky and lake were dove gray, as was my mood. There is a particular aloneness in staying behind not because you want to, but because you can't keep up. At least I had two treats: a beer Matthew gave me on the bus and some *droë wors* (dried meat sausage) we got when Brian discovered a South African store at our pee stop.

I opened the big window that looked out on Lake Lough Gill. The cool air smelled of moss and pine. I reclined on the couch. Then Edward, who works at St. Angela's, walked past my window. I needed a wedge to keep a heavy internal door open. I got up to ask if he had any extra door stops. He said he would bring me one. But instead of walking off to get it, he stayed to tell me that he too writes, and how he loves Tolkien, and how the first and second world work. How he believes in ginger and turmeric, but not in mindfulness. How he minds his dreams. I listened while shifting my weight from one leg to the other. When he paused, I took the opening and said, "I don't have much energy. Please excuse me, I am going to sit down."

I didn't sit for very long before there was a knock at my door. There stood Edward, with two door wedges in his right hand, one wood, one plastic. And in his left, a bottle of local beet juice.

"Here," he said, handing me the juice, "This is good for your energy." I inspected the bottle of crimson juice. He could tell that I was pleased by his gift and proceeded to tell me of other things that might help with low energy. I told him that my lack of energy is a result of a terminal illness. He didn't quite know what to say, so he said everything that came to mind. I listened until the end of his story about bee stings that stimulate the lymphatic system that can cure many illnesses. Then I excused myself again.

The next day the beet juice went into my smoothie. But my body was not used to this quantity of root vegetable essence. During dinner on Saturday evening it felt like someone was stitching my stomach lining to my diaphragm. I couldn't finish my dinner. Back at home, my travel companions heard about my discomfort and told me to wait outside their dorm. Donna came back with ginger tablets, Rachel with peppermint oil. The oil mixed with water soothed me to sleep. As I settled, the corners of my mouth turned upwards.

### First-hand lake, second-hand sea

On Sunday morning Rachel walked me down to the lake. It was warm enough to swim! Donna held up a towel to create a changing room for me. I was for this water like a desert was for rain. I couldn't get in quickly enough. But the ragged rocks bit into my feet, soft from city shoes. I was afraid I'd fall. Sienna offered her flip flops. Matthew and Carlow took my hands and walked with me until I could lower myself into the bosom of the lake to be caressed by the silky water. There are no words for how much I love to swim.

Carlow walked me all the way out of the lake and then returned to swim some more. I hurriedly dried myself, as I still needed to pack before we left. Again Matthew helped me carry my things to the bus.

The lady at reception said, "Please come back!" I

replied, "I definitely will." It was not quite a lie. My heart really wanted to. But my body, this body, is dying. Then Edward came up to shake my hand, his green eyes sparkling, and said confidently, "I will see you again, Hanna."

Part of our group was staying behind to go swim in the ocean—something I longed for just as much if not more than swimming in the lake. But I didn't have the energy. I dragged myself to the back of the bus. I wanted to come back. I wanted to swim in the Atlantic and have dinner at Brian's place, then take the train back to Dublin. I wanted to, but I could not. Brian came to hug me goodbye. A small storm of loss rumbled through me and spilled into public view. Rachel came and sat beside me, put her hand on my back, and offered me a tissue.

On Monday, back in the air-conditioned class-room of Trinity College, Teddi took a seat next to me. She is one of the people who stayed in Sligo to visit the ocean. When the reading ended, she handed me a tiny see-through shopping bag. In the bag were three shells she picked up at the beach. I held one to my ear and I heard the song of the sea. My heart swelled and tingled like bubbles on a breaking wave.

That night I woke up in the wee hours unable to return to sleep. I reached for the large shell. It fit snugly in my hand. I rested my thumb in the smooth opening. My phone played the sound of the ocean and I imagined myself being carried.

## Circles of care

On our second-to-last evening, we had a student reading at Books Upstairs. The shop greeted me with that good old bookshop smell. To my right was a table with all the classics bound in colorful fabric. My fingers itched for them, but I walked past and up the wooden stairs to a small salon style space with tall windows overlooking D'Olier Street.

Each student got to read for up to four minutes. I felt proud of the people around me. When it was my turn, I put on a tiny mic and ramped up the volume on my little speaker. I used my ventilator to help me take generous breaths after reading each paragraph. The audience had a printout so they could follow along. My friend Marc bought me the Lady-Gaga-style mic and formatted the printout. Many friends contributed for me to afford the ventilator.

To be heard even as my words become mush and voice recedes is to be validated as a whole person.

After the reading we went to a pub. Tess got up and offered me her seat. Brian put half a pint of Guinness beside me. One of the mentors that I hadn't met pulled her chair close to mine. She told me about a friend of hers who had passed away from ALS. We proceeded to have a lively conversation that helped me feel seen and heard, even though I was using mostly a pen and paper and occasionally my phone to communicate. When she got up, she wrote down her email address and said, "Please. Please email me. I am here for you in any way I can be."

After the excitement of the evening wore off and the beer settled in, we realized that the kitchen had already closed. It was past my bedtime (I had been really good at getting to bed early!) but my hunger drove me into the street with the rest of the crew. The only place close and open was an American diner!

After a burger and fries we made our way back to Trinity, our fingers sticky with ketchup. It was after 11pm. I was grateful for Brian's arm that held me steady as we walked through the bustling street, over bumpy pebble stones and alongside a man clearly high on something. We arrived at Trinity where many of our group stood gathered under the hundred-foot-high stone constructed bell tower. Our program said that there would be a rose moon reading at midnight, but I had no hope of being awake then. I was barely awake as I stood there, so I headed for my bedroom.

It was, and is, difficult for me to discern how much I can do without overextending myself. Once in my room and ready for bed, I felt a longing for the gathering. So I zipped my coat over my pajamas, slipped the room key into my pocket, and went out to find them. The group of writers had formed a circle under the tower. Inside that was a smaller circle made of fresh cut roses, and in the center were candles.

I arrived at a special moment, I could tell. The circle opened and drew me in. Later I heard that moments before my arrival the group offered prayers and wishes for my health. Standing there, braided into the ring, I was given the candle and the opportunity to set an intention for the new moon. All I could think as I was being held so tenderly by this group was, "Thank you, thank you, thank you."

### The kindness of life in loss

After check-in for my flight home, the lady at the counter ordered a wheelchair. I waited in the designated area. The gentleman who came to get me arrived too soon.

"May I have three minutes to say goodbye to my friend, please?" I asked.

"Of course," he replied. "Take your time."

Amelia, a dear old friend from South Africa, picked me up after the residency, and we had a fabulous four days on the west coast of Ireland. Both of us grew up in a world with no tolerance for tears. And now, here we were at Dublin airport about to say goodbye whilst both of us knew this might very well be the last time we saw each other. My tear tide was already rising.

"Well," she said, "I think we can do what we were taught to do. We sweep the fact of your illness under the rug and pretend it doesn't exist."

"Let's do that," I replied. We leaned into a long hug.

I said, "Come visit in Pittsburgh."

She said, "See you when you travel through London again."

We disengaged from the hug, and I sat down in the wheelchair. James, the gentleman helper, wheeled me off.

I felt empty, as if the tide of tears had receded leaving only a vacuum pulling at my throat. Waiting for the elevator doors to open, I saw Amelia out of the corner of my eye. She had followed us. She stood there, blue Café Nero coffee cup in hand, smiling. I smiled back.

Then the doors opened, and James pushed me into the small space. I looked back over my shoulder and Amelia appeared within view. She waved, I waved. As the stainless-steel doors slid closed, Amelia kept moving to hold my gaze until the door snipped our eye contact like scissors and the escalator started to ascend. The corners of my mouth curled down and tears began to roll. I held back a sob.

When the doors opened again, I used my sleeve to wipe my eyes. I felt a warm hand on my shoulder followed by, "Are you okay, miss Johanna?" It was James' voice.

> But really it was
> the kindness of life,
> meeting me once again.

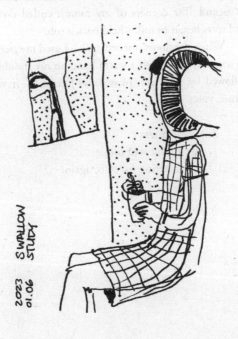

SWALLOW
STUDY

2023
01.06

# Bright green box

After my swallow study, the doctor tells me that his job is to see to it that I die of old age, and we both laugh, knowing I won't make it to forty-eight. He hands me a clear plastic tube, three inches long with a blue bubble attached to one end, and shows me how to put it where my tongue makes the 'k' in cookie. He tells me I should use my tongue to press the tube against my palate for three seconds, then rest before doing it again. If I repeat this five or ten times every other day, it might slow my tongue from turning into stone.

Bright green box

Then he asks if I received the EMST, and I vaguely remember yet another masked woman at the ALS clinic handing me a bright green box, showing me how to use the respiratory strengthening device inside, how to force the air out of my lungs. Three days a week I should blow five times, rest one minute, and repeat that three times. I diligently packed the damn green box in my suitcase to use when I travel, and it has followed me, unopened. This morning it sits on my dining room table, reminding me that I am dying and that I am not doing my best to keep living.

I push the box aside, noticing how my fingers curl in like a bunch of bananas, and now I feel guilty for not stretching them as the occupational therapist instructed. But with the table cleared, I do a stretch the physical therapist showed me—five reps of twenty-second holds, seven days a week—so I don't get a frozen shoulder: frozen, immobilized before its time,
the time it takes
for ALS to paralyze
enough voluntary muscles
for me to die,
before my time,
for a lack of trying.

# A dying girl goes
# to grad school II

January 2024

Dear Carlow companions,
I'm so glad to join you for the January writing residency. I am writing because for the first time in my life, I am attending grad school in an actually disabled and dying body. Going on a writing retreat with a terminally ill person might be new for you too. So it's bound to be awkward, but maybe I can share some things that will help us both get a feel for what it may be like.

### I AM NOT IN CONTROL

On the ALS functional scale, I have lost 60% of my abilities. That's a lot of body no longer functioning well! I'm like an old phone who might suddenly run out of battery life mid-workshop, please excuse me. My legs seem to miss running and will break out in a tremor at the weirdest times. Just welcome it.

### I NEED FULL TIME CARE

A beloved friend, Laurie, is flying in from Montana to be my companion. She is cut from the same cloth as Rachel Walton and will fit right in. I'll be leaning on her and if we need more support, we will ask you.

### I LOOK AND ACT DISABLED

Which means that even though I feel like a songbird inside, I am disabled. I even have the parking sticker. In my able-bodied life, I found it trying to relate to disabled folks, and you might too. If you feel the urge to pity me or be overly nice and helpful, please go get a coffee and drink it slowly until you feel ready to try seeing me in my wholeness.

YOU WILL SEE LITTLE OF ME

This disease is a jealous bastard and has me breathing with a BiPap for twelve hours each day. It requires me to stretch daily, so my limbs don't turn into kettle-fried crisp. And eat, OMG, I eat with a tongue that moves like a geriatric snail. So on a good day I will join you for three hours. I will not be able to generate much writing during the residency.

I AM MUTE

I communicate by writing on a board, which Laurie will read. I miss talking! And I hate being talked at. I invite you to share silence with me. If I write on my board and invite you with a gesture to read, please read aloud to bring my voice into the room, so I know I have written legibly and you have understood. When you want to know my preference, please ask me questions I can answer clearly with a yes or a no. If you ask two questions at once, I cannot respond and be understood. For example: Don't ask "Would you like coffee or tea?" Please ask, "Would you like coffee?" Then wait for a reply, and if I say no, ask if I would like tea.

## THE PARALYSIS IS AFFECTING MY LIMBS AND CORE

It is like the dial of gravity keeps turning up and my limbs seem to be stuck to surfaces. I heard yesterday that I am approved for a portable electric wheelchair which I don't know how to drive yet! I hope to get it before the residency. You can also bet that I will be the slowest mover. Please excuse me if I roll in late!

## MY LUNG CAPACITY KEEPS LESSENING

Any respiratory disease (a common cold, a flu, a mysterious sniffle) can land me in the hospital and I will not recover to this level of functioning again. This is a source of stress for me. I want to be in community, be loved and held and not get ill. My neurologist has made it clear that I must mask at all times and invite others close to me to do so, and to up their hand washing game. Please be on the side of my safety. If we share a writing space and you are able, please mask up. If you or someone in your household has a respiratory infection, please keep your distance from me. It's hard for me to ask, because I am a hugger-bear, but please be conscious of transferring cooties—don't touch me without consent.

Because of this I will not join you for dinner, which is a sadness (I love hanging out, I love good food) and a relief (because I am gross).

I AM GROSS

After your speech muscles go, your swallow functions
follow. So be glad we are not sharing a meal! And
even if we don't dine together, my gross warning
persists: I am no longer able to manage my saliva
well and I can choke by swallowing my saliva (and
disrupt your reading). With lungs that can't cough so
well, there will also be excessive throat clearing. I'm
not trying to get your attention; I just have phlegm
in the wrong place.

MY EMOTIONS ARE RIGHT THERE, READY TO SURFACE

Don't be alarmed if I cry. Don't be scared if my
laughter sounds like a donkey in labor or if I vocalize
frustration in a moan. Part of dying is being vividly
alive also. I feel stripped of my filters. Please just be
in the moment with me. There is nothing to fix.

Despite all this and no makeup, I am still a beautiful badass and I am excited to be with and learn from you as we keep writing, shifting, breaking, righting, and remaking ourselves and this world.

With so much love,
Hanna

# I was angry when
# you picked me up late

because I really had to pee, and unlike you who can whip out your penis and aim it at a urinal, I wait for the disabled bathroom (a popular place to poop), then I maneuver the wheelchair in at the right angle, park, power off so I don't accidentally knock my caretaker over, then I need help to stand up, pull my panties down, lower myself onto the seat and only then can I pee; also, you texted "on my way, stay in a warm place" three minutes before you were supposed to be here but by then there was a) a disabled entrance with a broken key-card and b), three slopes between us and that "warm place," and I was already starting to slide down the slope—damn this icy weather—and I didn't want to career all the way onto Fifth Ave as I almost did on Saturday, and besides a nice lady was talking to my caretaker, asking, "Does she need help?" as if I am not a fully functioning human being—even though I can't manage to keep my saliva in my mute mouth, I can be in conversation you know (if you help me take my mitten off and hand me my board to write on)—but I digress, I was angry because we were waiting in that merciless wind, gusts pushing Canadian cold right up into our eyeballs turning my ALS-infested extremities into metal, metal with nerve endings which is to say they resounded with pain and then, then wetness mizzled from the sky, and it wasn't even pretty like snow, just half frozen sky-sweepings and when, finally, you arrived and my furious eyes disappeared between my ill-fitting mask and my oversized hat, I couldn't even tell you how pissed I was, forced instead to steep in my misery, though I really wanted to tell you, as you are the only man who can hear my anger.

# Is life worth living in the furnace of suffering?

This is not the first time I ask this question. Before becoming ill the question would burn for a few days. Then life's wonder would pour into me and the thought would recede in a smolder.

But a diagnosis like this is different. Your exile and suffering will increase till you are eclipsed by it. Days after diagnosis I meet with my therapist. Through prior months of tests, the two of us have held ALS as a possibility. But now it is my future. I ask, "Is life worth living with ALS?"

My therapist says, "Can we pause this inquiry and not come to a conclusion prematurely?" Her gaze holds me with tenderness, her voice a stability in this mauling mess.

Later a friend asks, "Do you consider taking your life so you can be spared this suffering?"
I pause.

What do I want?

What is that place
between fighting and acceptance?

What is the gap between my fear-
filled projection and the wonder I am
unable to imagine?

I don't know.

I tell my friend I won't kill myself.

I say,

"I owe it to myself to see what happens."

41

# The week in numbers
### Mon 24 Feb - Fri March 1

15 caregivers coming in, learning, loving, leaving.

One x-ray, one blood work, one steroid injection

Five times vitals taken

13 hours of meetings with Medical providers:
2x nurses, pulmonologist, shoulder specialist,
x-ray technician, phlebotomist (blood work),
physical therapist, occupational therapist,
massage, nutritionist

1.5 hours writing

209 hand written instructions or
requests for explanations

4,600 ml of feeding tube formula

2 boxes of tissues for spit and tears

One birdfeeder busted up by squirrels

86 occurrences of laughter

3 trips to pharmacy

5 nights of (not really) sleeping in a pain storm

300ml Tylenol (pain relief) and 45ml of oxy

3 deliveries of beautiful food

Countless small acts of care

33 hours of sunshine

0 minutes of standing in the sunshine

# Gratitude to
# my donor

Dear Donor,

Thank you for what you have made possible for me. In November of last year I started to develop symptoms of bulbar onset ALS. Coming from a healthy family and having been well for most of my life, the five months between symptoms and diagnosis was a black night of swimming in an anxious sea. When I was diagnosed and given two years to live with the prospect of a slow and unstoppable demise, I fell into questioning whether life was worth living. But a disease like ALS does not permit long spells of despair, because there remains a ridiculous amount of work to do to make sure you have medical coverage, the equipment you need, accessible housing, etc. I felt like this darn thing consumed me.

The program director's call in April, a month after my diagnosis, and the possibility of enrolling in the MFA opened a much-needed avenue through which life returned to me. I had been yearning for the structure and support of Carlow University's MFA program, but it wasn't financially possible for me. Being white and educated already, I didn't feel like I deserved a scholarship. There are people who need it more than me. So I want to thank you for what you made possible for me.

Where this terminal illness asks me to end the career I felt so passionate about, you gave me a new beginning.

Where this curbs my mobility, you helped me get out and travel to Ireland!

Where this shrinks my world of engagement with others, your generosity opened a community of writers to me.

Where this confines me to a chair, through my writing I am going to wonderful and frightening places.

Where this can take over my life, the monthly deadlines have given me permission to prioritize and claim my creative practice.

Where this can make me feel like deer turd, like a good-for-nothing writer, the monthly mentorship and feedback is building my belief that my voice is worthy of being heard.

Where this has taken away my ability to speak, this program is giving me voice.

Where this illness will ultimately take my life from me, my words will be companions to those I leave behind.

Yesterday I cried, not spoons or cups, but buckets of tears. A friend asked me what I was feeling. I wrote, "How would you feel if you could no longer speak, and are losing your ability to lift your limbs, chew and swallow, breathe without support or travel home to be with family?"

He paused and said, "I'd feel afraid."

I wrote on my board, "I am terrified."

He held my hand. We breathed together. Then he asked, "Can I tell you what helps me when I feel afraid?" I nodded yes.

"I remember that I am loved."

Thank you for your love that is a lifeline in this dark time. I am beyond grateful to you for choosing to invest in me, and to Tess the director for seeing me and introducing me to you.

I respect the fact that you are anonymous. But if you ever want to meet in person, please know that I would love that.


Wishing you so much wellbeing.
Hanna

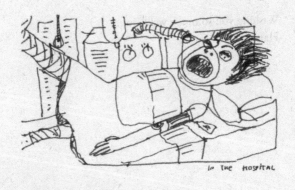

IN THE HOSPITAL

# Tearing of my worlds

If I could draw, I would pull up the picture of the evolution of man—the one with the ape growing taller and more human-like until it becomes an upright modern man. I would start with an upright woman, walking with confidence. Then she'd be slightly hunched over, then walking with a cane, then there's more curve in her back as her hands lean on a walker. Then I would round her back more, contort her hands and feet, strap her arms to an upright walker. Then three wheelchairs. The first is a loaner from the hospice. The second a portable electric chair, then the real-deal chair complete with headrest, mounted speech device and "sip and puff pipe" for breathing support (the one I am writing

49

from now). Finally the woman would recline on a hospice-supplied hospital bed. If I was feeling morbid I would end by drawing flowers growing strong from the worm farm I had become.

In June of 2024, a year after our Ireland residency, my friend brings me my phone.

"Look!" she says, "Donna has sent you pictures from Dublin!" My body tightens into a fist, bracing against the feeling of loss.

The watermelon-colored roses in Donna's photo bring a memory to my body. Just last year I got up from my writing bench to bury my nose in that same rosebush. I long to be there again in writing heaven with my people. That memory and that longing clash with my current condition. I experience a pulling apart—the world moving out of my reach while the self I know recedes into a mute motionless shallow-breathed being.

It feels as if I have built my life on a fault line and the earth is cracking open under my bare feet, pulling and splintering the pine floor boards, snapping the timber frame like match sticks, ripping the siding of my shelter apart. My eyes burn with dust, my lungs grasp for oxygen amidst particles of paint and plaster. I can't keep steady and start to slip out of my home into the moist earth below.

The contrast between my life now and my life in Dublin a year ago illuminates how slow dying tears my world apart.

Dublin: the sky holds the colors of the best sunsets all blended together. The ocean is quiet. Small waves lap against the concrete pier by the airport. The stillness of the water replicates itself in the waters of my body. This is our last sunset together before Amelia and I fly to our separate homes. It is summer solstice. From now on the days will only get shorter, like my life. Less light, less life.

A year later, the days grow long, but it is past equinox in my body. I sleep more than I am awake. My neurologist tells me I am in the advanced stage of ALS and gives me a hospice script. I struggle to reconcile my ambition with my reality. The best I could offer life yesterday was to shower and Zoom with my family.

Last year I flew on an airplane, and rode a bus on which James provided us with superb mental snacks. I walked carefully over the cobblestones and up the stairs to our reading without aid, enjoying the freedom to roam. I traveled to the west of Ireland and ferried across waves.

Now the plague of locusts has moved over the

51

lush field of my musculature, leaving lifeless tissue in its wake.

Last year in Ireland I sank my eager mouth into soft salmon and finished a pint of Guinness with glee.

This year at the Fourth of July cookout, I long for a burger. Photos show me laughing in my wheelchair, hooked up to something that looks like an IV drip. But it is plugged into a port on the left side of my torso, two inches under my breast. 90% of my food consists of factory made "complete meals" the color of cardboard, piped to my belly through a tube. If I want anything by mouth, I must ask someone to prepare and feed me finely-diced food. Any liquids—yes beer and coffee too—must be thickened and fed to me. And please don't forget my bib and tissues for drool.

Last year in Ireland and as I came home to Pittsburgh, I felt woven into life. Every day held an adventure, a reading, a group dinner, a boat ride to Inishmore, a canoe trip down the river. I felt a sense of belonging to multiple communities, landscapes, places and bodies of water. I felt a freedom I took for granted.

Now I feel how disability stitches you down in place and covers you up. I often feel invisible and blind. Blind because of my mute mouth, and hands that rest on my lap like a marionette with cut strings. I can't reach for my phone, call a friend. I can't discover events or invitations serendipitously. It feels like I am forgotten. Even though more people think and pray for me than any time before, I feel as though I have slipped out of being seen as part of life. I have received two invitations to events in three months. It's lonely to be homebound, despite the garland of caring community.

I miss being in the world, a world made for me. And when I finally spend thousands to rent an accessible van so I can push into life with friends, I find myself stuck. Stuck at the side of the pool because the chair that lowers cripples into the water is broken. Stuck just outside the dance floor, because they forgot there is a step barring me from rolling onto it. Stuck on a wheelchair lift, missing my partner's daughter's last primary school concert, waiting forty minutes for the technician to arrive and to stop the incessant beeping and deliver me from the cage.

Last year I returned from Ireland and was embraced by my beloved. I spent the night at his home and woke with my head resting on his shoulder, my hand on his chest, held by his. I've often said to him, "This is a favorite place."

For the last ten months my lack of ability has kept me from being at my partner's home. No more reading bedtime stories with kids lying on top of us, hands scratching backs and stroking hair while Minas the cat purrs among us.

Now at night I feel like a surfboard packaged for international travel. I lie with silicone stickers and sheepskin on my bony bits to cushion against bedsores and water blisters. I have sleeves on my arms to prevent chafing. Five pillows prop up unmoving limbs. My scapula is tucked, arms pulled down, fingers spread and curled around a pillow. Ventilator mask on, TENS unit pulsing. A cherry-red cocktail of three pain meds has been pushed through my tube (they taste like a children's party if I burp). I lie motionless. A magnetic pull burns in my body, this limp and pained body wanting only one thing—to be held by my beloveds. But I am held hostage by gravity.

I am becoming too weak to stay on the second floor bedroom with the double bed. The hospital bed my neurologists ordered is a single bed. It feels like such a cruelty that those who are leaving life or losing beloveds are left to sleep alone.

After my alarm goes off I have twenty minutes for yoga before I need to get ready for breakfast at The Buttery. Rachel gave me a yoga mat the color of coal, printed with a constellation of stars. I roll it out and settle in, legs up the wall, my foam yoga block under my sacrum. When I'm done with my back routine, I sink the weight of my upper body into the warrior one pose. I feel the tension in my hips soften. I have always been a body for motion, be it downhill biking, long swims, hikes or yoga. At least it will be a while before ALS wrestles yoga away from me.

My hands were the first part I couldn't stretch on my own. The occupational therapist, working in a siloed system, prescribed hand exercises that took an hour a day. As if I wasn't dying on multiple fronts. But our group hunkered down and stretching my hands became part of every day. Around our January residency I could no longer exercise my arms by myself.

ALS is a heartless landlord, relentlessly evicting me, tearing my belonging apart, sending me and my naked arse into the streets. The worst days are when I have no more fight. When I slip out of all shelter, the mud parting between my crumpled feet, black waters rising, swallowing me completely, and I feel nothing.

# Five stars

Throughout my life, when my father and I would look at the night sky, his right hand would lift and his pointer finger would lead my eyes to two familiar stars.

"See those two stars?" he would ask. "They are the pointers." Then he would start at the top pointer, draw a line to the second star, and extend the line until it met the constellation of the southern cross. From there my dad would curl his fingers but keep his thumb and pinky extended to measure the length of the cross. Then he would extend the length four-and-a-half times along the axis of the cross. His pointer finger would reappear.

"There," he would say with satisfaction. "If you draw a line from this point straight down to the horizon, you will know where south is. And if you know that, you can find your way."

When my body slammed into the reality that I might have ALS, it was dark night and black waters all around. My familiar constellations were gone. My eyes darted around for way-finders. I needed to build something to steer me through this crushing passage.

I don't remember the sequence, only that I turned to those who have gone before me. I listened to a young man in Brooklyn. He was mute, so his cousin was reading his words. His diagnosis dragged him into a deep depression. It was only after his feeding tube operation (which in my experience felt like being badly beaten up) that he regained a sense of purpose and will to live.

I read a blog by a woman my age. Upon her diagnosis she went on a quest to be healed. She spent the better part of her health chasing down a miracle, and died without finding one. I had at least ten people who believed they had a cure for me, if.... If I believed this way, or thought that way, or attended this course, ingested that.... Despite the fact that they had no experience with ALS, and not referencing the work thousands of experts were doing to find a cure.

Having had my magical thinking crushed too

many times, and having sat under the deadening weight of depression myself, I discovered...

## My first star

DO WHATEVER IT TAKES TO COME INTO
AGREEMENT WITH REALITY, TO PLAY THE HAND
YOU WERE DEALT, DESPITE YOUR WISH TO CHUCK
IT INTO THE BLENDER AND WATCH THIS DECK
OF DEVASTATION DISAPPEAR INTO SMOKE.

## Second star

I listened to an interview with Stephen Hawking (I didn't watch, because I find the sight of him terrifying knowing he is now a mirror of me). He said, "I focus on what is possible." Not wanting to will myself into being a person that always smiles and finds the silver lining, I mixed his sentiment with what I knew I needed. Star two:

GRIEVE, WITH ABANDON, ALL YOU ARE
LOSING. PAUSE, AND WHEN YOU'RE READY,
FOCUS ON WHAT IS POSSIBLE.

### Third star

My dear friend had been a babysitter for Leah, the founder of the organization called "Her ALS Story." She encouraged me to have a conversation with Leah. It was my first real-life encounter with someone living with ALS. She was compassionate and inspiring. She was using her experience to build community for young women with ALS and advocating for legislative change.

When we ended our conversation she said, "I'm so incredibly sorry this is happening to you." I choked with tears. I heard myself say, "ALS is not only going to happen to me. I am also going to happen to ALS." The star there:

I WILL USE EVERY OUNCE OF AGENCY AVAILABLE TO ME TO RESPOND TO THIS BOA CONSTRICTOR WITH CREATIVITY AND PUSH MORE LIFE INTO THE WORLD.

### Star four

My most reliable source of wisdom is when I become quiet and open to the vast luminosity that some call God or Spirit. What I find there still challenges me. It says quietly and as clearly as a traffic sign, "Trust this." I don't know what to make of that intellectually, but my bones feel it. The words straighten my spine.

I keep this close to my heart together with the prayer, "Please show me how."

One night I listened to Andrea Gibson talk about their journey with terminal cancer. They were asked a question from the deep: "Can you love your cancer?" Hearing this, I started to weep uncontrollably. How does one trust and even love the beast that will destroy me? I don't know. But, as I have quoted Peter Block many times during facilitations, "The answer to how is yes." It is time to drink my own medicine. The fourth star:

> LEAN TOWARD TRUSTING
> AND LOVING WHAT IS.

## The fifth star

What I didn't mention and what you wouldn't know if your gaze hasn't traced the southern cross, is that there is a faint star between the arm and foot of the cross. That one, as my colleague and bestie Marc reminds me, is for the fifth star:

> STUBBORN JOY.

Now, extend the long axis four and a half times. Where that line ends, draw another line straight down to the horizon. South is there, even though you can't see it. Orient yourself the way migrating birds do towards the destination calling you. Now move, readjust course, move again, pause, feel for direction, find the magnetic pull and move again. Remember that you are not alone in this darkness, trust in the help, both seen and unseen.

You can make this journey.
Home is waiting for you.

# About the author

Hanna's life has centered on the possibility that people can become more able to co-create a thriving world.

Hanna grew up in apartheid South Africa, and came to the US in 2009 to study design. Shortly after, she embarked on a mission to transform herself and share what she learned with others, "so we can get good at the collective work of healing, repairing, and re-weaving."

Hanna has co-hosted dozens of spaces of transformation—gatherings of change leaders, student cohorts, and entire organizations. She has been an artist, a dancer, a writer, and performed improv on stage.

In March of 2023, Hanna was diagnosed with ALS, a degenerative neuromuscular disease that slowly robs the body of its functions. She has committed her remaining time to writing, adventuring with her family, and being in her beloved community.

Follow Hanna's story and work by visiting okaythen.net/voices/hanna-du-plessis.

# More from Hanna

**COMING WINTER 2024**

*A good girl gets lost and free and found and sick*
All her life Hanna has grappled with questions of control and freedom, power and love, othering and belonging. These vivid, emotional, heartfelt essays create a gravity well of invitation for readers to walk deeply into these questions for their own lives and their own communities. Plus, more of Hanna's cheeky illustrations!

**COMING IN 2025**

*Just beginning to live: the ALS essays*
(Working title) Everything Hanna has written from inside her experience with ALS. An articulate companion for those who are personally connected with this disease, and a rare, raw revelation for those who are not.

**The author wishes to thank...**

Tess Barry

"The donor" (see page 44)

Faculty, staff and fellow students in the Carlow University Creative Writing MFA program, and at Trinity College Dublin

Geeta Kothari, Sarah Shotland, and Marc Rettig

Her family

The "Care Force" community of care

Thanks to Team Gleason for my wheelchair-enabled grad school experience, and the co-pay for my gaze-tracking device. Also the ALS Association, and so many other organizations and caring professionals.

Without you none of this would be possible. You bring me to life!

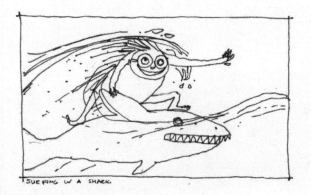

SURFING W A SHARK.